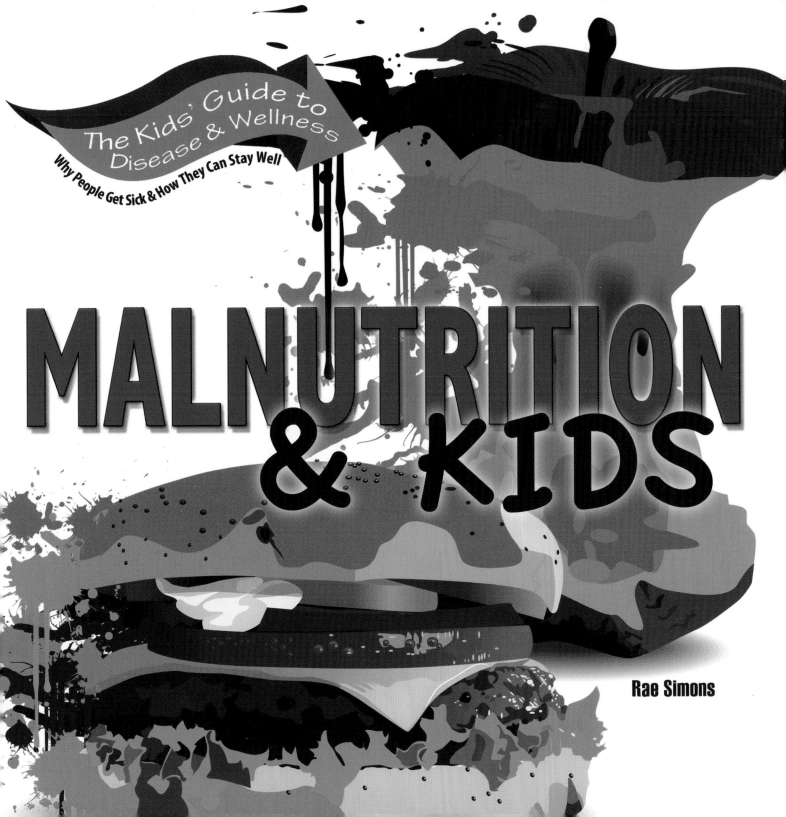

The Kids' Guide to Disease & Wellness
Why People Get Sick & How They Can Stay Well

MALNUTRITION & KIDS

Rae Simons

The Kids' Guide to Disease & Wellness:
Why People Get Sick and How They Can Stay Well
MALNUTRITION & KIDS

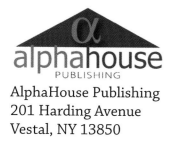

AlphaHouse Publishing
201 Harding Avenue
Vestal, NY 13850

First Printing

9 8 7 6 5 4 3 2 1

ISBN: 978-1-934970-19-5
ISBN (series): 978-1-934970-11-9
   Library of Congress Control Number: 2008930677

Author: Simons, Rae

Cover design by MK Bassett-Harvey.
Interior design by MK Bassett-Harvey and Wendy Arakawa.

Printed in India by International Print-O-Pac Limited

 An ISO 9001 Company

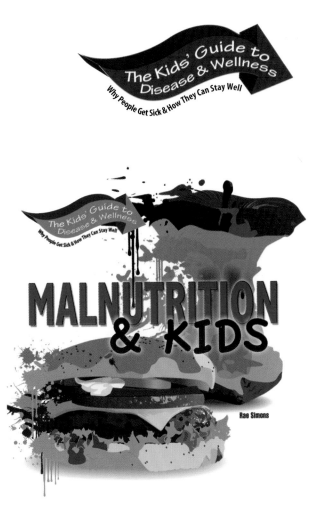

The Kids' Guide to
Disease & Wellness
Why People Get Sick & How They Can Stay Well

MALNUTRITION & KIDS

Rae Simons

By Rae Simons

Series List

Bugs Can Make You Sick!

Pollution Can Make You Sick!

Cancer & Kids

Why Can't I Breathe? Kids & Asthma

Things You Can't See Can Make You Sick: Viruses and Bacteria

Kids & Diabetes

What Causes Allergies?

Malnutrition & Kids

AIDS & HIV: The Facts for Kids

Immunizations: Saving Lives

Introduction

According to a recent study reported in the Virginia Henderson International Nursing Library, kids worry about getting sick. They worry about AIDS and cancer, about allergies and the "super-germs" that resist medication. They know about these ills—but they don't always understand what causes them or how they can be prevented.

Unfortunately, most 9- to 11–year–olds, the study found, get their information about diseases like AIDS from friends and television; only 20 percent of the children interviewed based their understanding of illness on facts they had learned at school. Too often, kids believe urban legends, schoolyard folktales, and exaggerated movie plots. Oftentimes, misinformation like this only makes their worries worse. The January 2008 *Child Health News* reported that 55 percent of all children between 9 and 13 "worry almost all the time" about illness.

This series, **The Kids' Guide to Disease and Wellness**, offers readers clear information on various illnesses and conditions, as well as the immunizations that can prevent many diseases. The books dispel the myths with clearly presented facts and colorful, accurate illustrations. Better yet, these books will help kids understand not only illness—but also what they can do to stay as healthy as possible.

—*Dr. Elise Berlan*

Just The Facts

- Food contains different nutrients that give us the energy we need and make our bodies work like they're supposed to.

- Carbohydrates give your body energy. There are two kinds of carbohydrates: simple and complex (which are healthier).

- Protein builds muscle cells and keeps our nerves healthy.

- Fat is found in a lot of foods. We need some fat, but too much can be unhealthy.

- Vitamins are found in fruits and vegetables and keep our bodies working like they should. We also need small amounts of minerals, which are found in the soil that plants grow in.

- A balanced diet includes enough of everything that your body needs in the right proportions.

- Malnutrition happens when someone doesn't have a balanced diet. Obesity is a kind of malnutrition. Poverty is often connected to malnutrition.

- Processed food is not as healthy, since many of the nutrients have been removed during processing.

- While fast food is quick and easy and tastes good, too much of it can be bad for you.

- Malnutrition can cause diseases like anemia and scurvy.

- Countries around the world are working to end poverty and malnutrition.

What Is Nutrition?

Nutrition is what we get from the food we eat. It's the "good stuff" in food, the things that are listed on food labels.

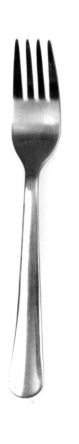

Nutrition Facts

Per 1 meal

Amount	% Daily Value
Calories 0	
Fat 0 g	**0 %**
Carbohydrate 0 g	**0 %**
Protein 0 g	

Not a significant source of saturated fat, trans fat, cholesterol, sodium, fiber, sugars, vitamin A, vitamin C, calcium or iron.

It's the part of food that gives our bodies what they need to function—to live and move, to think and breathe, play and work. Without nutrition, we wouldn't survive for very long!

Words to Know

Function: work, perform normally.

Why Does Your Body Need Food?

The food we eat contains different types of nutrients (the materials that supply us with nutrition). These nutrients include calories, carbohydrates, fats, proteins, vitamins, and minerals. We need some of all these. Our bodies are healthiest, have the most energy, and work their best when they have a balanced diet made of different foods that contain all the nutrients.

Words to Know

Balanced: being in a healthy and steady state where there is not too much or too little of anything.

Did You Know?

Calories are the units used to measure the energy you get from food. Your body needs a certain amount of calories every day. (Most people need between 2000 and 3000 calories, depending on their size and energy level.) When you eat more calories than your body uses, the extra calories are stored as fat.

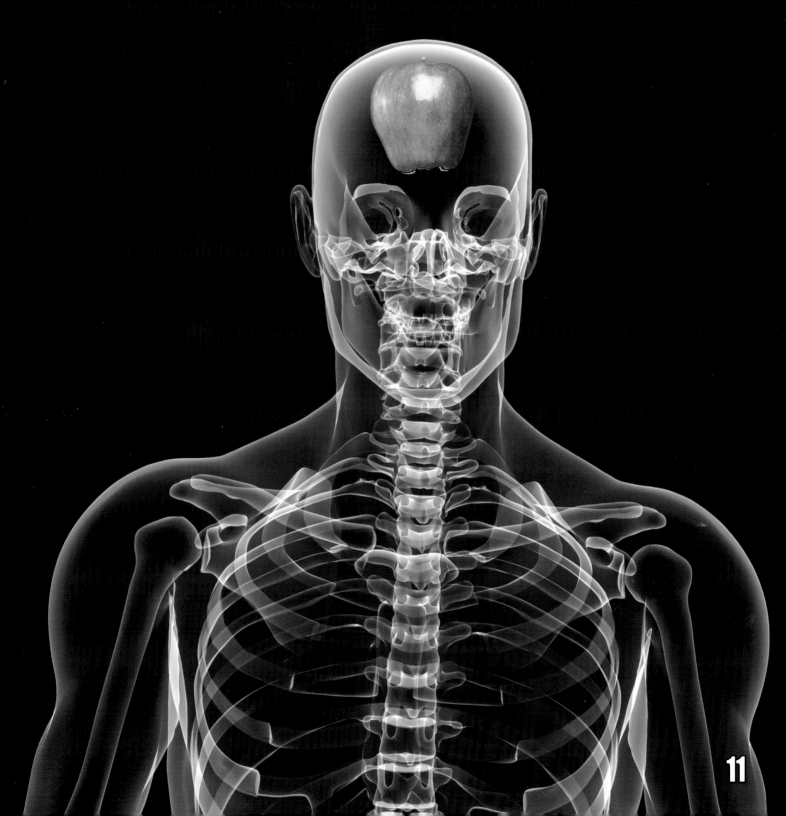

11

What Are Carbohydrates?

Carbohydrates give your body energy. They're your body's main fuel. Carbohydrates can be refined (simple) and unrefined (complex). Refined sugars (like those found in soft drinks, snack foods, and white bread) have already been broken down by food processing; in other words, machinery has removed all the bits of fiber from the food.

Words to Know

Fiber: the coarse, indigestible material found in plant foods that helps your intestines move along food.

Complex: having a more complicated structure.

Did You Know?

Bread, cereal, pasta, rice, candy, cookies, and cakes are all carbohydrates. Whole-grain breads, cereals, and brown rice are all complex carbohydrates.

Often, sugar has been added to the food, instead of being a natural part of it (as is the case with fruit and vegetables). Your body has to work harder to get the energy from unrefined carbohydrates. These more complex carbohydrates are better for you. Good nutrition requires more complex carbohydrates and as few refined carbohydrates as possible.

What Is Protein?

You need protein to build muscles and keep your nerve cells healthy. Protein is found in animal foods: meat, cheese, eggs, and milk. It's also found in some plant foods, such as beans, nuts, tofu products, and peanut butter. When you eat a balanced diet, it's easy to get the protein you need.

Words to Know

Tofu: a food often made from soybeans.

Not everyone eats as much protein as they need, though. Junk foods like chips, cookies, and other snacks are low in protein. For many people who live in the developing world, foods that contain protein are expensive and less available than other foods.

What Is Fat?

Fats are found in oils, meats, and dairy products. Junk foods have lots of fat! A high-fat diet is unhealthy. People who eat a lot of fat are more apt to be overweight and have a variety of diseases, including heart disease.

But fat isn't ALWAYS a bad thing.

Words to Know

Absorb: take in.

Insulators: materials that separate things that conduct electricity.

16

We need fat in our diets. The right kind of fat in the right amounts is good for you. It provides calories that give you energy. Fats are needed to absorb some vitamins. Fats are the building blocks of hormones, special chemicals that give directions to your body. And fats are the insulators for your body's nerve cells.

17

What Are Vitamins?

Vitamins are found in fruits and vegetables. Three of the most important vitamins are:

The B vitamins (found in beans, peas, and whole-grain foods) that help your body make energy.

Vitamin C (found in oranges and other citrus fruit, tomatoes, cabbage, and red and green peppers) that helps your skin and muscles keep healthy. It also helps cuts and wounds to heal and helps you ward off illnesses.

Vitamin A (found in carrots, pumpkin, yellow squash, apricots, and eggs), which is good for your eyes.

Your body doesn't need as large quantities of vitamins as it does proteins, carbohydrates, and fats, but if you don't get enough of the right vitamins, you will not function as well mentally and physically. Since your body can't make the vitamins it needs, you have to get them from food. That's one reason why experts recommend we try to eat 5 servings of vegetables a day. Each vitamin has a role to play to keep you healthy, and vegetables are a good source of vitamins.

What Are Minerals?

Minerals are the chemicals found in metals and in the soil. It may seem strange that your body needs something like iron (the same substance that's used to manufacture steel for cars and machinery) or copper (found in coins and cooking pots)—but it does! Your body needs only very tiny bits of minerals like these, but those tiny bits are important for good nutrition.

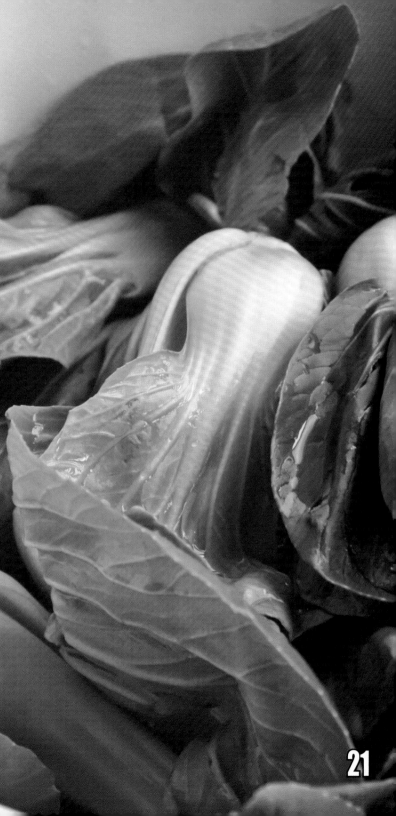

You don't eat coins or metal pots, of course (and too much of many minerals could be bad for you), so how do you get minerals inside your body?

First, plants take in minerals from the soil—and you get those minerals from eating plants. Iron, for example, which keeps your blood and brain cells healthy, comes from green leafy vegetables. Animals also eat the plants, and the minerals enter their bodies, so you can get some minerals —like calcium that's good for your bones and teeth—from eating meat and drinking milk.

What Is a Balanced Diet?

A balanced diet includes just enough of all the nutrients your body needs. Around the world, different countries have different ways to think about a balanced diet. In Canada, good nutrition is pictured as a rainbow, with each food

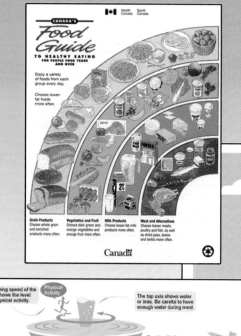

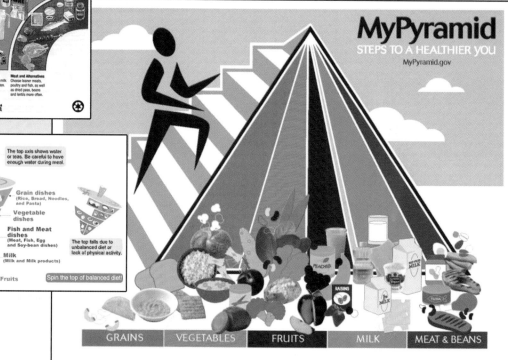

group a different colored stripe. The United States uses a pyramid to show what good nutrition should look like. Each stripe is a different food, and foods with higher calories are at the top of the pyramid, where the stripes are more narrow (showing that you don't need as much of those foods). Meanwhile, in Japan, a balanced diet is pictured as a spinning top, with each layer of the top a different type of food.

Words to Know

Calorie: a unit for measuring energy.

What Is Malnutrition?

Malnutrition is when our bodies don't get all the nutrients they need. A person with malnutrition is more likely to catch diseases.

Malnutrition can also affect brain function and eyesight. Your body organs (like your heart, lungs, and liver) won't work as well. Even the cells of your body—the very tiniest pieces of you—will not be able to work well if you don't give them the nutrients they need.

If a child has malnutrition, he may not grow as tall or weigh as much as would be normal for other children his age. If a pregnant woman is malnourished, the fetus within her may not develop normally.

Words to Know

Fetus: a developing human before birth, while it is still inside its mother.

What Causes Malnutrition?

Malnutrition exists all around the world, in rich nations as well as poor ones.

People may have enough money for food and still be malnourished because the foods they choose to eat don't give them the nutrients they need.

Meanwhile, people who live in poverty are often malnourished because they simply don't have enough food to eat. The foods they do have often don't offer them a balanced diet.

Words to Know

Poverty: the condition of being poor: not having the money or other resources for basic needs such as adequate food and housing.

Poverty in the Developing World

Children in many parts of Africa and Asia are hungry every day. Their families have very little money for food. Because of droughts and wars in the regions where they live, there may not even be enough food grown.

Words to Know

Drought: a long period of dryness when it doesn't rain.

What food these families have is often whatever is cheapest, usually carbohydrates such as the rice the child is eating here. These foods offer calories for energy, but very little protein, vitamins, or minerals.

Poverty in the Developed World

People also live in poverty in the world's developed nations. Homelessness is a growing problem in many cities. A person who has only a cardboard box for a home can't very well prepare nutritious

Words to Know

Developed: countries with plenty of businesses and industries where many services are available to the people who live there.

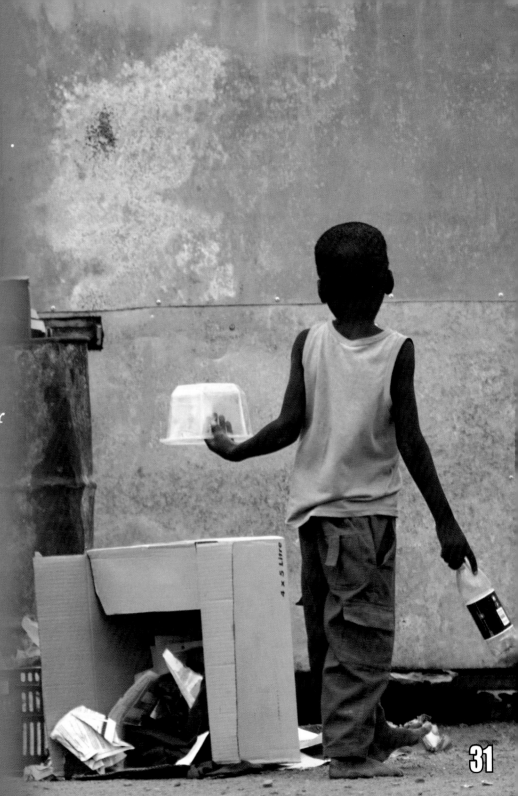

meals for himself. What food he does have may come from the garbage in a dumpster. Children growing up in poor families often don't have the nutrients they need. Even though grocery store shelves are lined with nutritious foods, poor families may be only able to afford the carbohydrates that cost less, like white bread, potatoes, and pasta. These fill you up, but they don't give you as many vitamins, minerals, and proteins.

Eating Habits

People who live in poverty may have fewer eating choices—but many people can choose what they eat and yet still choose to eat foods that don't offer them good nutrition.

Words to Know

Traditionally: having to do with a customary pattern of thought or behavior.

Unprocessed: not treated in any way (such as cooking, freezing, or adding chemicals).

Even fifty years ago, most people ate homecooked meals—but a lot has changed since then. Many women (the ones who traditionally prepared meals) work outside the home now, and families depend on food shortcuts. Hotdogs make a fast and easy meal—but they don't give you the same nutrients that fresh, unprocessed meat would. At the same time, many of us have become very fond of sweet snack foods, like ice cream, soda, and cake. These foods used to be the "reward" for good nutrition, but now they're regular snacks in many homes. They fill you up with lots of calories but few nutrients.

Processed Food

Processed food has been cooked, canned, or frozen. Although these "processes" make it easier to move foods from place to place and keep them for longer periods of time, they also remove vitamins and other nutrients from the foods. Fresh peas are much better for you than canned ones!

Many packaged foods are also made from white flour. White flour has been ground very fine. All the brown bits of fiber have been removed from it. Unfortunately, vitamins and minerals are found in those brown bits. Foods like the white bread shown here, as well as packaged cookies and other desserts, are not as nutritious as foods made from whole grains.

Did You Know?

Not all brown bread is better for you. Some brown bread is just white bread with food coloring added to it! Read the food label on the package. Whole-grain breads will have more fiber. Whole wheat or whole meal will be listed as their first ingredient.

Fast Food

ASK THE DOCTOR

My mother says I should quit eating fast food. Is she right?

A: Well, you should at least try to eat fast food only once in a while. Give yourself a limit, such as once or twice a month. Having an occasional fast-food meal isn't going to be the end of the world, but be careful not to let yourself fall back in the habit of eating too much of it too often. You don't need the fat, salt, and calories—but your body DOES need fresh fruits and vegetables (and you probably won't find them at a fast-food place).

Fast food is a growing trend around the world. It's quick and easy, and most people think it tastes good. With so many people in a hurry, it's a convenient way to grab a meal. Kids are especially fond of fast foods, partly because these foods are especially made to appeal to young people.

Unfortunately, fast food also has many drawbacks. One of the biggest is that these foods are high in fat and calories—and low in nutrients. The meal to the left, for instance, includes white bread (which we've already discussed), beef and bacon (both high in salt and fat), and french fries (high in fat and salt again). There are also a couple of leaves of iceberg lettuce, which are mostly water with very little else. The only food item in this meal that offers some vitamins is the tomato slice. That measly little slice, though, isn't going to get you far toward the 5 vegetables a day you need to be healthy.

Fast food may taste good—but if you lived on fast food, you'd probably also be suffering from malnutrition!

Words to Know

Convenient: suited to one's comfort and needs.

What About Vegetarians?

Vegetarians don't eat meat. Some vegetarians do eat fish and dairy products, but the most strict vegetarians (often called vegans) only eat plant products.

If you're a vegetarian, you can still eat all the nutrients you need to be healthy.

ASK THE DOCTOR

Is being a vegetarian healthier for you?

A: Vegetarian diets have many things going for them from a health standpoint: they're usually low in fat, for example: Some scientific studies suggest that vegetarians live longer than people who eat meat. However, you can eat healthy and eat lean meats—like poultry (chicken or turkey) and fish. Being a vegetarian is a personal choice that for many people is based on moral reasons; they feel it is wrong to kill animals, or they feel that eating only plants is a more responsible choice from an environmental standpoint.

Vegetarians must eat different kinds of vegetable proteins to make sure they get enough. For example, they need to eat beans with rice—or a rice cake with peanut butter. Soy is a good source of protein for vegetarians. Most protein bars and protein powders use soy protein, casein, or whey as their base, which are all complete proteins. Whey, however, is a milk product, so if you are a vegan, you may want to avoid whey products.

Words to Know

Strict: precise, exact, "hard-and-fast"

Whey: the watery part of milk.

How Does Malnutrition Hurt You?

When you don't get the nutrients your body needs, every cell in your body pays the cost.

Words to Know

Cell: an important unit of every living organism's body.

Malnutrition affects your bones, your organs, your blood vessels, your nerves, and your brain. Each part of your body needs nutrients in order to do its job. If a part of your body isn't getting what it needs to work well, you will not feel as healthy or strong. You may not grow as much. You may even get sick.

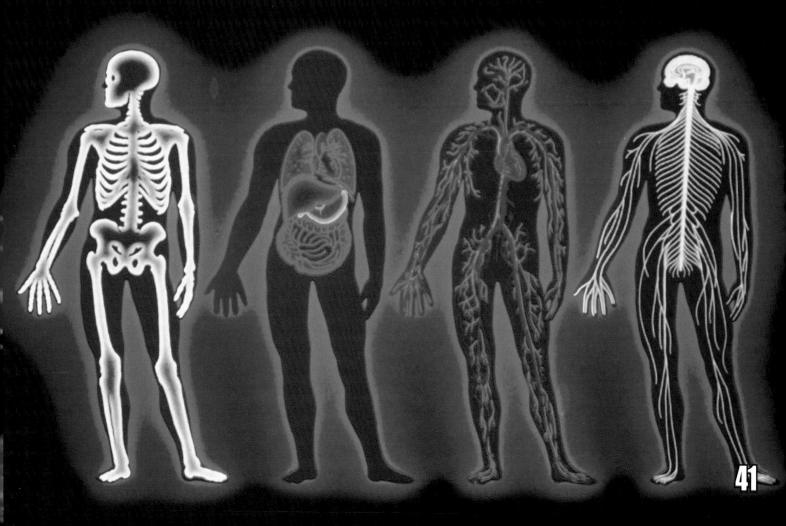

Growth & Development

Good nutrition is especially important when our bodies are developing. Children who do not get the nutrients they need don't grow as well. They will also have other problems. For instance, getting enough iron is especially important for children between the ages of six months and two years. Some countries add iron to baby foods.

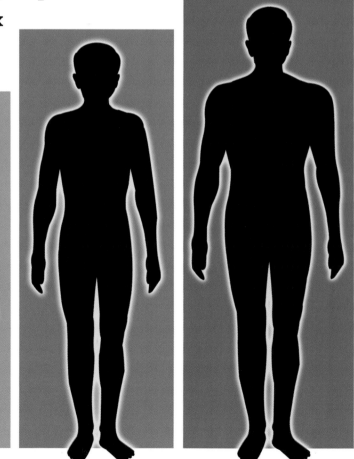

Prenatal care is very important also. Pregnant women need good nutrition more than ever, but for people living in poverty this is hard to achieve sometimes. As many as 18 million low birth-weight babies are born every year because of their mother's malnutrition. These children tend to get sick more, not grow as much, and have learning problems.

Words to Know

Prenatal: before birth (during pregnancy).

43

Your Brain & Your Moods

What you eat also affects your moods. For instance, when you eat lots of sugary foods, you may feel happy and excited at first, as the sugar rushes through your blood to your brain. Pretty soon, though, your blood sugar will drop. The same thing happens if you skip breakfast or other meals. When you have low blood sugar, you often feel tired and cross. You may get upset more easily. That's why it's important to listen to your body's messages and give it regular, well-balanced meals that include both protein and carbohydrates.

Words to Know

Function: the role or job of someone or something.

The B vitamins are especially important for your brain's function. Whether you're taking a test or playing a game, these vitamins help your brain do the very best job possible. They're found in cheese, milk, green vegetables, and whole-grain foods.

Energy Levels

To have the energy you need for school, home, and play, you need plenty of healthy carbohydrates—foods like bread, cereal, pasta, and rice. Your body breaks down carbohydrates into simpler sugars. These sugars are your body cells' "fuel." Its what gives the cells energy to do their jobs.

Did You Know?

Scientists have found that kids who eat breakfast pay attention better in school, read and do math better, do better in gym class, and get in less trouble.

And when your cells are doing their jobs, you have the energy you need to do all the things you want to do. That's another reason why it's important not to skip breakfast or other meals. When you do, your cells are like cars running on empty. They don't have the fuel they need—and you'll feel the difference.

So include carbohydrates in every meal. And remember, whole-grain, high-fiber breads and cereals are much healthier for you than sweet donuts, cookies, or cakes.

Your Immune System

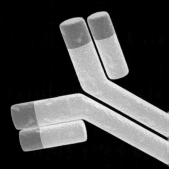

Your immune system is made up of all the parts of your body that help you fight off diseases and infections. Special cells in your blood attack and destroy germs (as illustrated on the page to the right). When your body doesn't get enough protein and vitamins, though, it can't make as many of these cells. This means that invaders—the germs that make you sick—are more likely to slip by your body's defenses.

Words to Know

Defenses: protections or shields against attack and injury.

48

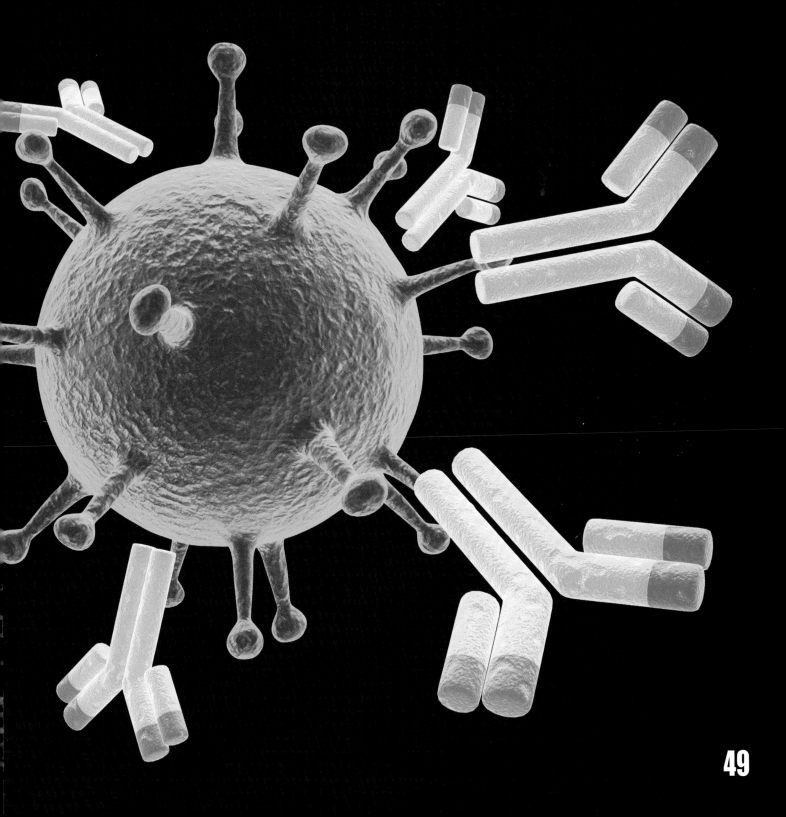

Diseases

Certain diseases are caused by not getting enough of specific nutrients. Anemia, for example, is often caused by not eating enough iron (found in red meats and dark green vegetables). Your body needs iron to keep your red blood cells healthy. Without enough iron, you don't have enough red blood cells to carry oxygen to your cells, and you feel tired and weak. Scurvy is another disease caused by a nutrient deficiency. Sailors used to get scurvy because, during their long sea voyages, their diets lacked fresh fruits (which contain vitamin C). Scurvy caused the symptoms shown in the man shown on the bottom of the next page. Some people still use "scurvy" as an adjective for someone who looks scary and disgusting. But people who had this disease really couldn't help how they looked!

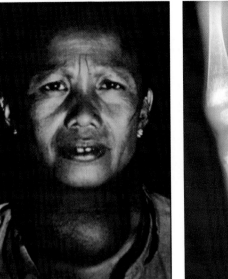
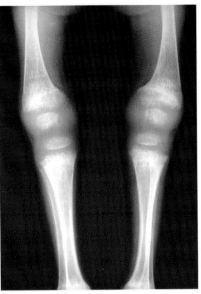

The woman to the right has a goiter, caused by a lack of the mineral iodine. The child's X-ray shows that he has rickets, a softening of the bones caused by a lack of the mineral calcium.

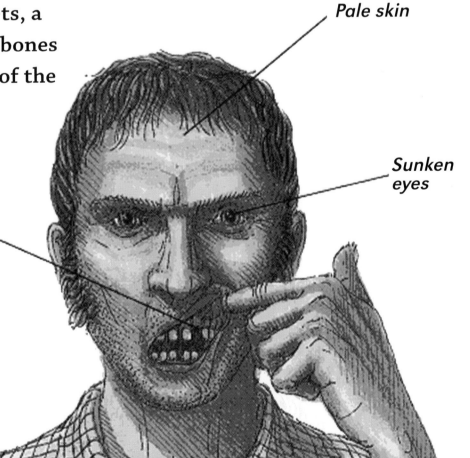

Pale skin

Sunken eyes

Loss of teeth

Obesity

You might think that obesity is just the opposite problem from malnutrition. But that's not the case. Many people who are obese don't eat a balanced diet. They eat lots of calories but not many nutrients. This means that their bodies store the extra calories in the form of fat, and all the while they're not getting the nutrients they need for good health.

Poverty often plays a role in this. Foods with lots of calories and not many nutrients (like fast food, white bread, pasta, and white rice) tend to be cheaper than foods with lots of vitamins and protein (like fresh vegetables, fruits, and meats). High-calorie foods fill you up without costing a lot of money. Unfortunately, they also make you fat without providing the vitamins, minerals, and protein you need for good health.

Many children and teens also eat these sorts of foods, not necessarily because they're poor, but just because they like them! Sugary snacks, french fries, burgers, chips, and cookies all taste good. They're easy to grab as an after-school snack (or for breakfast when you're running late). Because of this, more and more children and teens are overweight or obese. This can cause them health problems as they get older. And at the same time, their bodies are not getting the nutrients they need for good health.

Words to Know

Obesity: extra body weight that is dangerous to your health.

What's the World Doing About Malnutrition?

Words to Know

Organizations: groups working together to accomplish a common goal.

Obstacles: things that get in the way or keep something from happening.

Countries around the world have recognized that malnutrition is a big problem. They're working together to find ways to improve nutrition. The United Nations, an organization made up of most of the world's nations, is finding ways to help the world's people get the foods they need for good health.

One way to do this is to fight poverty, since being poor is one of the biggest obstacles to healthy eating. Education is another important weapon in the war against malnutrition. When people understand what good nutrition is—and why it's important—they're more likely to make healthy food choices. This kind of education takes place with both children and adults. It happens in schools and on televisions, on the Internet and on street posters.

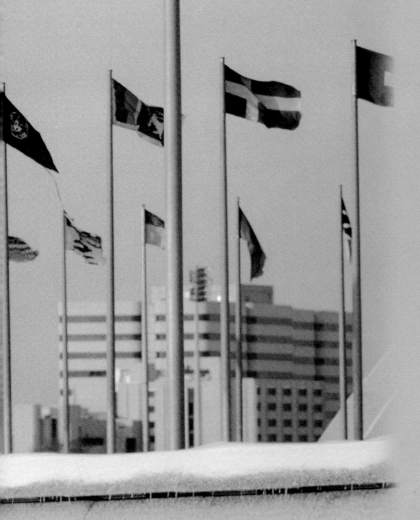

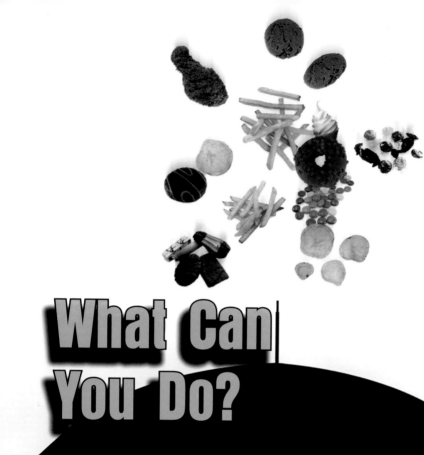

What Can You Do?

You can do something about malnutrition:

Make a list of healthy foods you like and that your family can afford. Try to eat foods from that list every day.

Help your family and friends understand how important it is to eat a balanced diet.

Words to Know

Whole-grain: grains that keep all their parts.

Remember to eat every day:

- fresh fruit and vegetables
- meat, dairy products, beans, or nuts
- whole-grain cereal, breads, pasta, and rice

Limit how many fatty, sweet foods you eat. Your body will thank you!

Real Kids

Tim Perkins was an ordinary kid who lived in Toronto in Ontario, Canada. His family wasn't rich and wasn't poor. They were pretty much like most of the other people they knew, except that both of Tim's parents were obese, and so was Tim. When Tim was nine years old, he weighed 185 pounds (84 kg). He and his family loved fried foods like french fries, fried meat, donuts, and chips. They didn't really like vegetables.

Tim never liked being teased about his weight, and he hated gym class because it was hard for him to run and keep up with the other children. But Tim is good at computer games, and he had lots of friends who shared his interest. He didn't worry much about being heavy.

But then Tim's father had a heart attack. The doctor told Mr. Perkins that if he didn't lose weight, he would probably have another heart attack—and this time he might die. That scared Tim and his family. His father went on a diet right away, and Tim and his mother decided to help him by eating the same diet. They stopped eating fried foods and started eating vegetables.

About this time, though, Tim started having chest pains too. His parents took him to the doctor right away. They were scared there was something wrong with his heart too.

It turned out, though, that Tim's chest was hurting because he has asthma (a serious breathing problem). The doctor said his weight was part of the problem.

Two years later, the Perkins aren't obese any more. They eat lots of fresh fruit and vegetables. They also eat lean meats and fish, lowfat dairy products, and plenty of whole-grain carbohydrates. They go for a walk every night after supper. And they feel great!

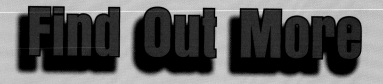

Find Out More

These books and Web sites will tell you more about malnutrition and good nutrition:

Health Canada
www.hc-sc.gc.ca/index_e.html

Hunger Notes
www.worldhunger.org/

MedlinePlus: Nutrition
www.nlm.nih.gov/medlineplus/nutrition.html

Millenium Campaign
www.millenniumcampaign.org/ site/
pp.asp?c=grKVL2NLE&b=185518

U.S. Government's Nutrition Site
www.nutrition.gov

Vegetarian Nutrition for Teens
www.vrg.org/nutrition/teennutrition.htm

World Health Organization: Nutrition
www.who.int/nutrition

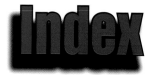 Index

Calcium, 21, 51
Calories, 10, 17, 23, 29, 33, 36, 37, 52, 53
Carbohydrates, 10, 12, 13, 19, 29, 31, 44, 46, 47, 59

Deficiency, 50, 51
Diet, 10, 14, 16, 17, 22, 23, 27, 38, 50, 52, 56, 59
Disease, 2, 3, 16, 24, 48, 50

Fats, 10, 16, 17, 19
Fiber, 12, 35, 47

Malnutrition, 24, 25, 26, 37, 40, 41, 43, 52, 54, 55, 56, 60
Minerals, 10, 20, 21, 29, 31, 35, 53

Nutrients, 10, 22, 24, 25, 26, 31, 33, 34, 37, 38 40, 41, 42, 50, 52, 53
Nutrition, 8, 9, 10, 13, 20, 22, 23, 32, 33, 42, 43, 55

Obesity, 52, 53

Poverty, 27, 28, 30, 32, 43, 53, 55
Pregnant, 25, 43

Proteins, 10, 19, 31, 39

Sugar, 12, 13, 44, 46, 53

Vitamins, 10, 17, 18, 19, 29, 31, 34, 35, 37, 45, 48, 53

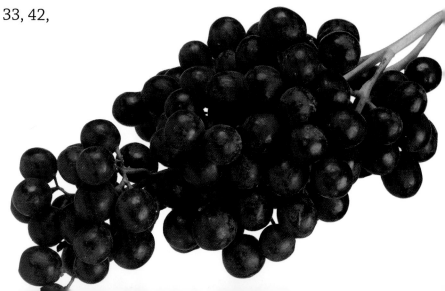

Picture Credits

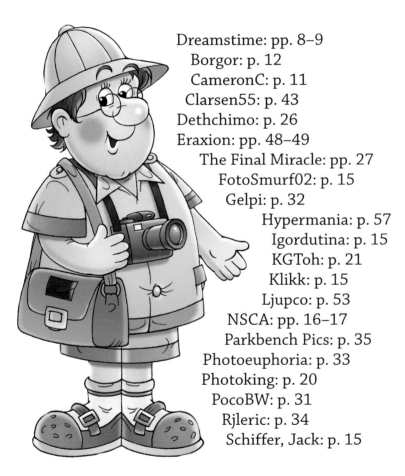

Dreamstime: pp. 8–9
Borgor: p. 12
CameronC: p. 11
Clarsen55: p. 43
Dethchimo: p. 26
Eraxion: pp. 48–49
The Final Miracle: pp. 27
FotoSmurf02: p. 15
Gelpi: p. 32
Hypermania: p. 57
Igordutina: p. 15
KGToh: p. 21
Klikk: p. 15
Ljupco: p. 53
NSCA: pp. 16–17
Parkbench Pics: p. 35
Photoeuphoria: p. 33
Photoking: p. 20
PocoBW: p. 31
Rjleric: p. 34
Schiffer, Jack: p. 15

Soupstock: p.p. 24–25
Volare2004: p. 29
FDA: p. 22
Health Canada: p. 22
Japan Ministry of Health: p. 22
Jupiter Images: pp. 13, 14, 18–19, 23, 29, 30, 36–37, 38–39, 40–41, 42, 46–47, 54–55, 56, 58–59
Life Resources: p. 51

About the Author

Rae Simons has written many books for young adults and children. She lives with her family in New York State in the U.S.

About the Consultant

Elise DeVore Berlan, MD, MPH, FAAP, is a faculty member of the Division of Adolescent Health at Nationwide Children's Hospital and an Assistant Professor of Clinical Pediatrics at The Ohio State University College of Medicine. She completed her Fellowship in Adolescent Medicine at Children's Hospital Boston and obtained a Master's Degree in Public Health at the Harvard School of Public Health. Dr. Berlan completed her residency in pediatrics at the Children's Hospital of Philadelphia, where she also served an additional year as Chief Resident. She received her medical degree from the University of Iowa College of Medicine.